D1384169

Photographic Case Studies in

▶ Neurology

Diagnostic Tests for the Practitioner

David J. Coffey, MD
Lawrence R. Jenkyn, MD
Kerri L. Wilks, MD

Section of Neurology
Dartmouth-Hitchcock Medical Center

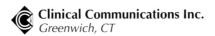

Clinical Communications Inc.
Greenwich, CT

Acknowledgement

The authors gratefully acknowledge Thomas Ward, MD, Harker Rhodes, MD, Laurence Cromwell, MD, and Pierre Bastianelli of the Dartmouth-Hitchcock Medical Center for their efforts in helping to make this publication possible.

Clinical Communications Inc.
81 Holly Hill Lane
Greenwich, CT 06830

ISBN: 0-9633775-2-3

This book is one in the series of *Photographic Case Studies* published by Clinical Communications Inc.

Publisher: *Corey Kupersmith, RPh*
Editorial Director: *Lois Gandt*

Printed in the United States of America

Introduction

The 1990's have been designated "The Decade of the Brain." Recent advances in diagnostic capabilities have been profound. The unique and challenging case studies presented here reflect the rapid advances that have taken place in the diagnosis of neurologic disorders.

This particular collection of unique photographs represents a broad spectrum of neurologic diseases that are encountered by clinical practitioners both in the primary care setting and in neurologic practice. The diagnostic photographs illustrate a variety of unusual diagnostic challenges in the form of clinical situations that physicians may not be likely to encounter in their everyday practice. While the patient history and neurologic examination continue to represent the foundation of evaluation, technical advances in diagnostic instruments have added greatly to the ability to more accurately diagnose neurologic disorders from the simple to the more complex.

The challenging illustrations enclosed represent a wide variety of possibilities, including physical signs; biopsies; radiographic, computed tomographic, and magnetic resonance images; and EEG, EMG, and CSF results. The clinician is challenged here to interpret clinical information as well as the results of diagnostic testing. We believe that this format is one that will sharpen your diagnostic acumen.

1 ▶ For 3 months, a 28-year-old woman experienced burning dysesthesias that spread up her right arm from the hand to the shoulder, axilla, and anterior chest wall. The arm was strong but clumsy. An MR scan was obtained.

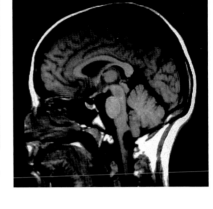

a) What are the three most likely diagnoses?

b) What medical treatment might be offered to reduce the pain pending surgery?

2 ▶ A 39-year-old convict was recently subdued and handcuffed after a skirmish with prison guards. He complained that the handcuffs were applied too tightly and that pain and numbness bothered him in the distribution shown.

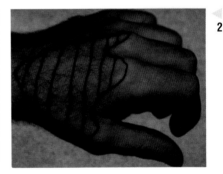

a) The most likely diagnosis is:
   1) Cheiralgia paraesthetica
   2) Carpal tunnel syndrome
   3) Cubital tunnel syndrome
   4) Thoracic outlet syndrome

3 ▷

4 ◁

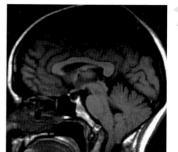

3 ▶ A 34-year-old woman fainted after a near-miss auto accident, and was subsequently noted to have generalized clonic activity of her arms and legs. A neurologic examination was normal. A CT scan was obtained.

a) Her CT scan after contrast most likely shows a(n):
1) Arteriovenous malformation
2) Glioblastoma
3) Meningioma
4) Calcified falx cerebri
b) After surgery, would you treat this patient with ethosuximide, carbamazepine, or clonazepam?
c) Clonazepam is contraindicated when the patient is taking which anticonvulsant?

4 ▶ A 57-year-old woman with a 1½-year history of intractable dry cough had a recent 3-month history of nasal regurgitation when drinking liquids. She also noted an occipital headache if she landed heavily on her heels when jumping. An MR scan of the head was obtained.

a) The responsible anatomic abnormality is most likely:
1) Hypoplastic cerebellum
2) Basilar impression of the brainstem at the cervicocranial junction by the odontoid process
3) Herniated cervical disc
4) Fibrocytic astrocytoma

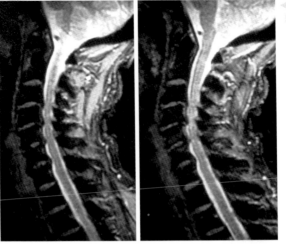

5 ▶ A 59-year-old man sustained multiple trauma in a motor vehicle accident 20 years prior. In the past 5 years or more he has become aware of a slowly worsening gait. On examination he had decreased reflexes in the upper extremities and increased reflexes in the lower extremities, with sustained clonus at both ankles. Plantar responses were extensor, bilaterally. There was a decrease in vibration sense in both legs. Serum B_{12} level was normal. There was no family history of a similar disorder. Needle EMG of lower extremity muscles revealed no acute or chronic denervation. The MR scan of the cervical spine is shown.

a) The correct diagnosis is:
- 1) Friedreich's ataxia
- 2) Combined systems deficiency
- 3) Spinocerebellar degeneration
- 4) Spondylitic myelopathy

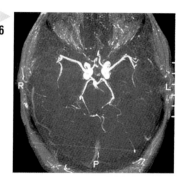

6 ▶ A 32-year-old woman returned for follow-up of a routine anterior cervical discectomy and was noted by the neurosurgeon to have a complete third-nerve palsy on the right. MR angiography was interpreted as negative.

a) In this situation, should a conventional cerebral arteriogram be obtained?

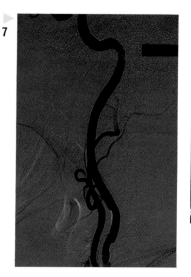

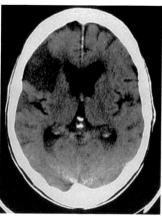

7-8 ▶ An 85-year-old woman with paroxysmal atrial fibrillation stopped taking her coumadin medication 7 days prior to dental work. Three days later, she developed a left hemiparesis and profound left-sided neglect. Carotid ultrasound showed an ulcerated plaque in the proximal right internal carotid artery with <70% stenosis. CT scan of the head is shown.

a) What does the CT scan show?
b) What are two possible mechanisms for this condition?

9 ▶ A 57-year-old man noted severe headaches after prolonged flexion of his neck at a computer terminal. Neck extension uniformly relieved the headache in a few minutes. An MR scan was obtained. Angiography was performed.

a) What disorders should be considered?

b) What does the MR scan demonstrate?

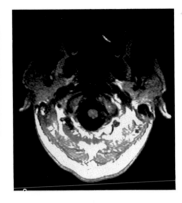

10-11 ▶ A 76-year-old man with a history of migraine, visual scotomata, and episodic musical auditory hallucinations presented with a severe headache, after which the scotomata persisted in his left visual field.

a) What abnormality is seen on his MR scan and cerebral angiogram?

b) What are the possible etiologies of the visual scotomata?

c) What are the possible etiologies of the auditory hallucinations?

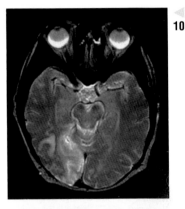

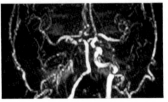

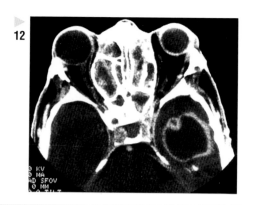

12

12-14 ▶ A 61-year-old man who lived reclusively and had avoided physicians for decades took a bus tour to northern New England to view autumn foliage. He checked into a motel, but aroused concern when by the fourth day he had failed to leave his room or pay his bill. He was found stuporous, jabbering unintelligibly, and was brought to the hospital. His examination was remarkable for a wide, flat nose, bilateral proptosis with divergent gaze, and extraocular movements present in all versions. Inspection of the nares showed that they were filled with nasal polyps. Polyps were seen extending below the uvula from the nasopharynx. His facial appearance was unchanged from that of his driver's license picture taken a year or so earlier. Neurologic signs included a mild expressive aphasia, pronator drift of the right upper extremity, flattening right nasolabial fold, and bilateral extensor plantar responses. A CT scan was obtained.

a) What is seen on the CT scan?

case continues

During the hospitalization, his condition deteriorated rapidly, with acute onset of fever, global aphasia, and right hemiparesis. Repeat CT scans of the head were obtained.

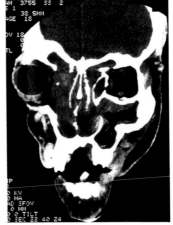

13

b) Does this image correlate with the clinical picture?

case continues

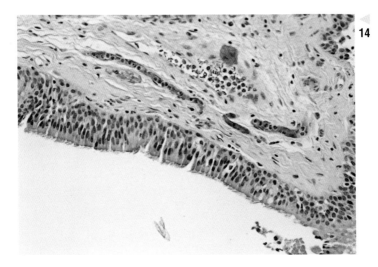

14

A subtemporal craniotomy with abscess drainage and anterior temporal lobectomy was performed. A biopsy photomicrograph is shown.

c) What is the tumor type?

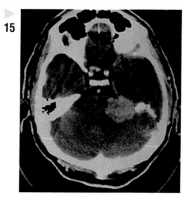

15

15-16 ▶ Seventeen years prior, a 44-year-old man lost hearing in his left ear. He presents now with ataxia, falling, and a reduced left corneal reflex. A CT scan was obtained.

a) Possible diagnoses include:
1) Acoustic neuroma
2) Meningioma
3) Metastatic tumor
4) All of the above
b) What is the pathologic diagnosis shown in the photomicrograph?

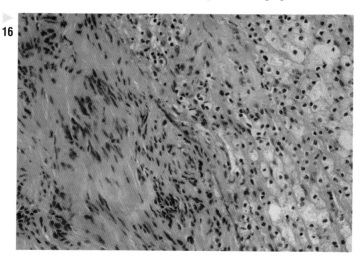

16

17 ▶ Slowly progressive burning dysesthesias of the hands emerged in a 41-year-old woman 1 year following whiplash injury to the cervical spine. Nerve conduction studies confirmed carpal tunnel syndrome bilaterally, but surgical decompression was unhelpful.

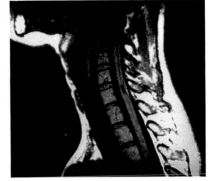

17

a) What does the MR scan of the cervical spine reveal?
b) What other symptoms and signs may evolve over time?

18 ▶ This patient had presented 4 years previously with ataxia but no tremor. Two years later difficulty with up gaze and then down gaze emerged. Presently, he has little control of his left arm which wanders uncontrollably at times, must throw his head in the desired direction of gaze to bring objects into central vision both laterally and vertically, and is wheelchair-bound by ataxia and slowness of movement.

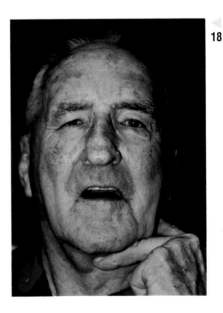

18

a) Diagnosis, please.
b) Is cognitive impairment a typical feature of this disorder?

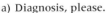

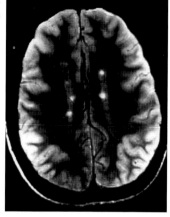

19 ▶ Six months prior a 23-year-old man had a 6-week episode of paresthesias in the right hemithorax, most notable after sexual intercourse or jogging. He now presents with an inability to adduct his right eye when looking to the left, but has no difficulty when accommodating to a near target. An MR image of his brain is shown.

a) The eye movement abnormality is called:
   1) Pendular nystagmus
   2) Opsoclonus
   3) Internuclear ophthalmoplegia
   4) Optic neuritis

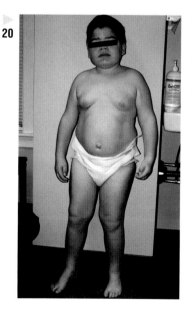

20 ▶ This 10-year-old child has Hunter's syndrome. Note the protuberant abdomen, flexion of the elbows, umbilical hernia, and widened hands and feet.

a) Which of the following is true?
   1) Mental retardation is present.
   2) Hepatosplenomegaly results from a buildup of mucopolysaccharide breakdown products due to deficient lysosomal enzymes.
   3) Affected children rarely live past the second decade.
   4) Dwarfism usually results by age 2 or 3 years.
   5) All of the above.

21 ▶ A 32-year-old woman presented with seizures in which there was suspension of consciousness without falling, raising of one arm with picking movements of the fingers, and turning of the head toward the upraised arm. An MR scan of the brain was obtained.

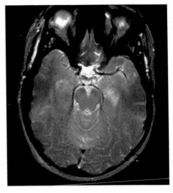

21

a) What is the seizure type?
b) What is the likely cause?

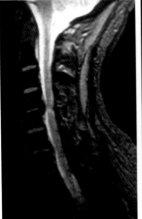
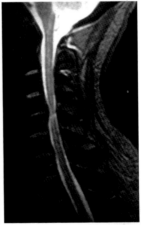

22

22 ▶ A 42-year-old man was carrying a tray of tools at work when he was struck by a heavy metal door. He developed pain in his right arm with considerable loss of coordination and inability to use the right hand unless he looked at it. He also complained of dysesthesias in the left lower extremity. Bowel and bladder functions were normal. Intrinsic right-hand muscle weakness, generalized hyperreflexia, bilateral ankle clonus, and bilateral Babinski's signs were found on exam.

a) What is the most probable diagnosis?

b) What does the MR scan of the cervical spine show?

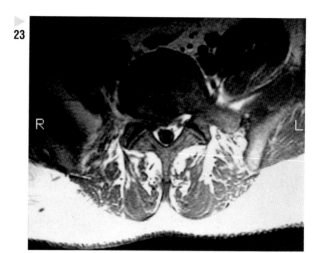

23 ▸ A 32-year-old man complained of 6 weeks of gradually progressive low back pain radiating to the right great toe. A CT scan was performed.

a) What does the CT scan show?

b) Would you expect this to improve on its own?

24 ▸ A 19-year-old with posttraumatic headaches heralded by right homonomous scintillating scotomata developed right-sided focal motor seizures with secondary generalization. These, too, were preceded by right homonomous scintillating scotomata. A CT scan was obtained.

a) What is the lesion seen on the CT scan?

25 ▶ A 37-year-old registered nurse had a history of multiple hospitalizations since adolescence prompted by abdominal pain, low back pain, and intractable headache. In each instance, workup was negative. She had been lost to follow-up for several years after she moved to the West Coast. Shortly after she returned East, her husband brought her to the emergency room in a state of diminished responsiveness.

a) What are the major concerns regarding her diagnosis at this point?

case continues

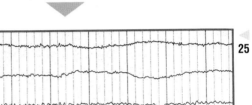

Examination revealed a thin, youthful-appearing woman lying supine with her hands folded on her chest. Her eyes were closed and she did not move when asked. Her facial expression suggested a frown. Her palpebral fissures were very slightly open and fluttered continuously. When the examiner attempted to open her lids, there was resistance and Bell's phenomenon was noted. When either hand was held above her face and dropped, it slipped easily past her face without striking it. With her eyes held open, gaze was convergent; pupils were equal, 4 mm in diameter, round, and reactive to direct and consensual light exposure. Optokinetic nystagmus to a striped band was noted in both directions. Gag and corneal responses were present. Deep tendon reflexes were normally reactive, and plantar responses were flexor. An EEG was obtained.

b) How would you interpret these findings?

c) What does the EEG show?

d) What risks remain and how is this patient best managed?

26-28 ▶ A 54-year-old school janitor with a 15-year history of benign familial tremor and a 5-year history of non–insulin-dependent diabetes mellitus was started on glyburide. Thereafter, he noted numbness and paresthesias in both legs and hands accompanied by acute, severe pain in both thighs and difficulty walking down stairs. The pain and proximal leg weakness cleared over 1 month, at which time his examination revealed only hyperesthesia to vibration and pin in all four limbs distally, greater in the legs, and 1+ deep tendon reflexes with absent ankle jerks. Nerve conduction studies were consistent with a diffuse sensory neuropathy of axonal origin. Amitriptyline was offered, and improvement in the dysesthesias was noted. Primidone improved his tremor.

a) What is the most likely diagnosis to explain his painful proximal leg weakness?

case continues

Ten months later the patient returned with several months of insidiously progressive weakness, fatigue, diaphoresis, and shortness of breath with any minimal work activity, episodic right upper quadrant and epigastric pain, and loss of voice with exercise. Gastrointestinal and cardiac workups were unrevealing. Creatine kinase (CK) was 239 IU/L (normal < 235 IU/L). Signs included 5/5 power proximally and distally (including neck flexors) without atrophy, fasciculations, muscle fatigability on repetitive contraction, or ptosis on sustained upward gaze. Needle electromyographic studies showed scattered chronic partial denervation in right upper and lower extremities, proximally and distally, consistent with diffuse sensorimotor neuropathy of axonal origin. Repeat CK was 228 IU/L; aldolase was 2.2 IU/L (normal = 2-7 IU/L).

b) What is the most likely diagnosis to explain these new signs and symptoms?

case continues

The acetylcholine receptor antibody (ARA) level was 0.51 nmol/L (normal < 0.03 nmol/L). Repeat ARA level was 0.64 nmol/L. Repetitive neuromuscular transmission studies were normal, failing to document an incrementing or a decrementing response at any rate of stimulation (from 1-50/s). A trial of pyridostigmine, 60 mg tid, was not helpful.

c) True or False: This man has myasthenia gravis.

d) True or False: This man has Lambert-Eaton syndrome.

case continues

An MR scan of the chest is shown.

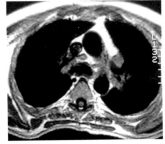

26

e) Why was the MR scan done?

f) What does the MR scan show?

case continues

Awaiting mediastinal biopsy scheduled for the next week, the patient developed a right Bell's palsy. Prednisone, 80 mg qd, was started the same day and the facial weakness resolved in 5 days. A chest CT scan obtained during steroid therapy was interpreted as normal and biopsy was deferred. The erythrocyte sedimentation rate (ESR) was 12 mm/h, serum Lyme titer was 0.95 (negative), and a carcinogenic embryonic antigen level was negative. Cerebrospinal fluid (CSF) was obtained under an opening pressure of 100 mmCSF and contained a total protein of 83 mg%; 10 WBCs/HPF (100% lymphocytes); a glucose level of 190 mg%; and negative Gram's and acid-fast bacilli stains, india ink smear, cytologies, VDRL, Lyme titer, and cultures. The myelin basic protein level was 1.6 ng/mL (normal = 0-4.0 ng/mL). Oligoclonal bands were positive.

g) True or False: This man may have multiple sclerosis.

case continues

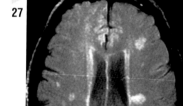

27

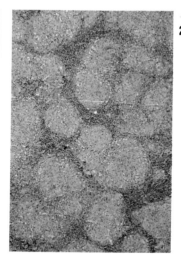

28

Steroids were tapered and 2 weeks later repeat MR and CT scans of the chest confirmed the presence of hilar adenopathy, increased in size over the first MR study. The MR scan of the brain (above left) revealed diffuse periventricular hyperintensities. These lesions did not enhance with gadolinium. Repeat ESR was 72 mm/h. Rheumatoid factor was positive. VDRL and RPR were unreactive. A third ARA level was elevated and a second serum Lyme titer was negative. Quantitative immunoglobulins and immunoelectrophoresis were normal. Visual, brainstem auditory, and posterior tibia somatosensory evoked responses were normal. Mediastinal biopsy was performed.

h) What does the biopsy reveal?

i) Does the patient also have myasthenia gravis?

j) Does the patient also have multiple sclerosis?

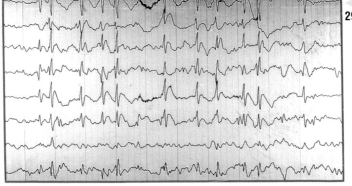

29 ▶ This EEG tracing was accompanied by unresponsiveness in a 9-year-old patient. No other behavioral changes occurred.

a) What is the most likely diagnosis?

b) Name two first-line anticonvulsants for this problem.

30 ▶ A 4-year-old boy had a 4-month history of progressive clumsiness, swallowing difficulty, and speech disturbance. He also developed double vision. A CT scan was obtained and was normal. His MR scan is shown.

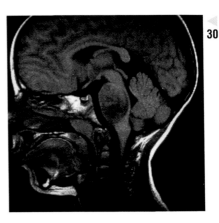

a) What is the likely diagnosis?
1) Cerebral palsy
2) Developmental delay
3) Pontine glioma
4) Bacterial meningitis

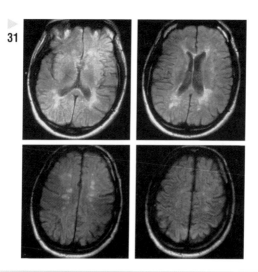

31

31 ▶ A 45-year-old journalist noted a partial left footdrop only after running. Initially, this came on after 3 miles but, more recently, it was evident at half a mile.

a) The MR scan is consistent with:

   1) Lyme disease   3) Multiple sclerosis
   2) Neurosarcoidosis 4) All of the above

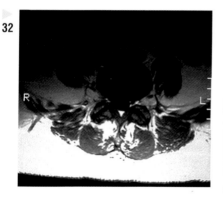

32

32 ▶ A 59-year-old man with several months of severe pain radiating from the buttock down the posterior right thigh to the anterolateral leg also complained of numbness in his right great toe. A lumbosacral MR scan was normal. A CT scan was performed.

a) What does the CT scan show?

33 ▶ A 34-year-old man fell into a hole at work 2 years prior, and has had low back pain with right leg pain ever since. He was noted by his company physician to have an absent right ankle jerk and an inability to step up to tiptoe on the right foot.

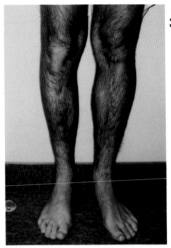

33

a) What is the likely diagnosis?
b) Would an imaging test have been valuable earlier on?

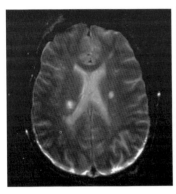 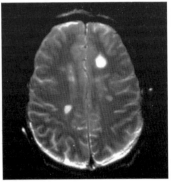

34

34 ▶ At age 16 years, this man had experienced a left hemiparesis that resolved after several weeks. At age 46 years, he noted sudden-onset vertigo, ataxia, and right-sided weakness. Signs included mild right hemiparesis, loss of position and vibration sense to the knees, and a positive Romberg sign. An MR scan after gadolinium was obtained.

a) What is the most likely diagnosis?

b) What does the MR scan show?

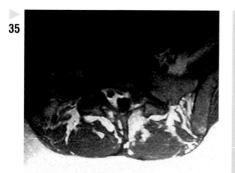

35

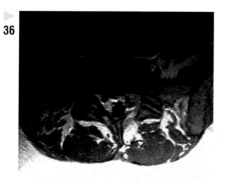

36

35-36 ▶ A 36-year-old woman who underwent a left L5-S1 discectomy/laminectomy 2 years previously now presents with subacute recurrent pain. She has pain in the low back, left buttock, and posterior thigh, with decreased sensation to pinprick in the lateral aspect of the left foot and loss of the left ankle jerk reflex. CT scans of the L5-S1 level without and with gadolinium enhancement are shown.

a) Most of the root compromise is by:
   1) Recurrent herniated nucleus pulposus
   2) Fibrotic scar tissue
   3) Lipoma
   4) Arachnoid cyst

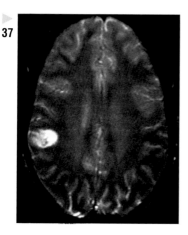

37

37 ▶ A 20-year-old college psychology major reported that she had "spells" of feeling "removed from her body." She had been driving at 65 miles per hour when her left foot began rhythmically twitching for approximately 20 seconds. EEGs in the awake and sleep-deprived states, and 24-hour ambulatory EEG were normal.

a) What does the MR scan show?
b) Does this explain her symptoms?

38-41 ► A 55-year-old woman underwent successful release of the right carpal tunnel 10 months prior to lovastatin therapy for hypercholesterolemia. After 4 months, she noted serious gait difficulties including inability to climb stairs or arise unassisted from a crouched position. She had fallen after prolonged standing, when her left leg became "shaky." Impairment of her sense of taste, weight gain, and tremulousness occurred during an empiric trial of prednisone for her leg complaints. Aching in the left calf and numbness and paresthesias in both feet had been present for several months as well. She was also taking nifedipine, losinopril, and cimetidine.

Findings included: fine action tremor in all four limbs, 3/5 neck flexor and 2/5 bilateral hip flexor power, Gowers' sign, 1-2+ symmetric upper extremity reflexes, 3+ right lower extremity reflexes, 1+ left ankle jerk, and absence of the left knee jerk. Plantar signs were flexor and there was no atrophy or fasciculation. All other signs, including tests of sensation, were normal.

a) This patient most likely has:

    1) A neuropathy
    2) A myopathy
    3) A familial neurodegenerative condition
    4) A defect in neuromuscular transmission

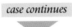

case continues

Blood studies revealed no evidence of anemia, infection, diabetes, renal or hepatic dysfunction, or altered electrolytes; cholesterol, 240 mg/dL; CK, 45 IU/L (normal = 21-215 IU/L); ESR, 14 mm/h; and serum lead, 7 mcg/dL (normal < 25 mcg/dL). Urinary lead, arsenic, and mercury excretion levels, an immunoelectrophoresis of serum, and acetylcholine receptor antibody levels were normal.

b) Does this information change your diagnosis?

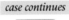

case continues

38

Muscle	Insertional Activity	Fibrillations	Positive Sharp Waves
L Tibialis ant	Increased	4+	4+
L Gastroc/sol	Increased	4+	4+
L Vastus med	Increased	4+	4+

Impression:
Widespread acute denervation in L3-S2 innervated muscles of the left leg suggesting diffuse motor neuronopathy (motor neuron disease).

Two weeks off lovastatin, the patient's neck flexor and right hip flexor strength returned to normal. Left hip flexor weakness persisted and physical therapy was prescribed for 1 month. At that time, the left quadriceps and hamstring muscles were weak at 4/5. Needle EMG studies in the left leg are shown. The right leg was intentionally ignored electromyographically.

c) What does the EMG result suggest?

d) Does this change your diagnosis?

e) Why were needle EMG studies not performed on the right leg?

case continues

Fasciculations	Firing Rate	Interference Pattern	Amplitude (max mV)
Rare	High	Reduced	2
Rare	High	Reduced	4
Rare	High	Reduced	5

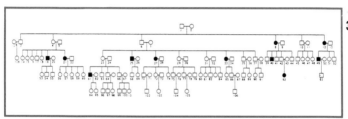

The patient's family history was strongly positive for amyotrophic lateral sclerosis (ALS) occurring in an autosomal dominant pattern (family members with ALS are denoted by solid symbols). The GM_1-autoantibody level was undetectable.

f) Does this change your diagnosis?

g) What test(s) would you order next?

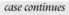

case continues

case continues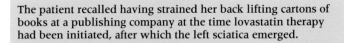

40   Specimen (a) Submitted:
MUSCLE BIOPSY-R Gastrocnemius muscle

PATHOLOGICAL DIAGNOSIS: Muscle biopsy with mild
neuropathic changes and ultrastructurally abnormal
mitochondria identified by electron microscopy.
See Comment

COMMENT: In most patients the ultrastructural
findings would suggest the possibility of a mito-
chondrial disease. However, we are uncertain how
to interpret them in someone with this patient's
background. We would welcome an opportunity to
examine pathological material from other members
of this patient's family. We would appreciate
clinical follow-up information on this patient.

The formal interpretation of a right gastrocnemius muscle
biopsy is shown above.

h) Does this change your diagnosis?

case continues

The patient recalled having strained her back lifting cartons of
books at a publishing company at the time lovastatin therapy
had been initiated, after which the left sciatica emerged.

i) Given the lack of improvement off lovastatin to this point (9
months later) what test(s) would you order next?

case continues

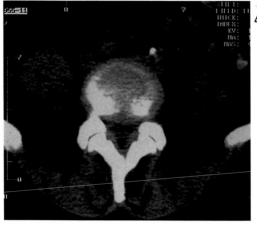

The lumbosacral CT scan is shown above. After 2 months, the patient's left leg was nearly totally paralyzed while the remaining three limbs were strong. Increasing sciatica responded to amitriptyline and oxycodone. After 3 additional months, weakness was clinically evident in the intrinsic hand muscles, bilaterally, in the right hamstring, and in the hip flexors.

j) What is your diagnosis now?

case continues

A second opinion at a major referral center resulted in repetition of the blood studies. In addition, Lyme titer and hexosaminidase α & β levels were normal. "Painful" transcranial magnetic stimulation of the brain failed to disclose motor conduction delays centrally. Bilateral arm and right leg needle EMG studies revealed significant denervation. DNA was obtained for a study of familial ALS and the patient returned home for terminal care.

42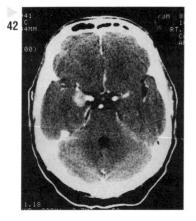

42-43 ▶ Recurrent, unexplained odors were noted by a 68-year-old man for over 5 years. A left hemiplegia resolved incompletely after surgery for the lesion shown in the CT scan and the gross pathology. Postsurgical administration of the same anticonvulsant on two separate occasions resulted in a persistent vegetative state (PVS) twice in 2 years. The PVS reversed each time upon discontinuation of the drug.

a) Diagnosis, please.
b) What anticonvulsant was most likely given postsurgically?

43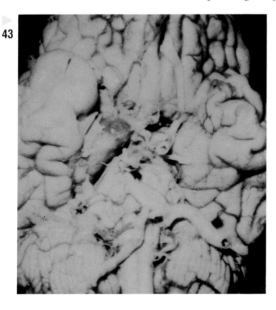

44 ▶ A 19-year-old girl experienced bilateral interstitial keratitis 3 months prior to a hearing loss in both ears accompanied by tinnitus, vertigo, and imbalance. Other signs included partial deafness, unsteady tandem gait, and inability to balance on either foot unassisted. The remainder of the neurologic exam, including appendicular cerebellar signs, was normal.

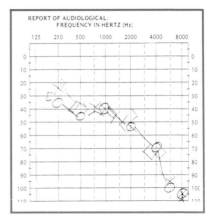

a) Diagnosis, please.
b) What is the treatment?

45 ▶ Over 2 months, a 31-year-old contractor developed incoordination of the arms and mild imbalance.

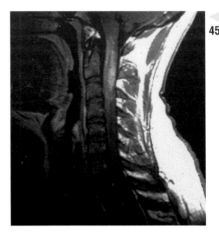

a) The MR scan most likely demonstrates:
  1) Multiple sclerosis
  2) Syringomyelia
  3) B_{12} deficiency
  4) A neoplasm
b) In which of these processes might enhancement occur after intravenous infusion of gadolinium?

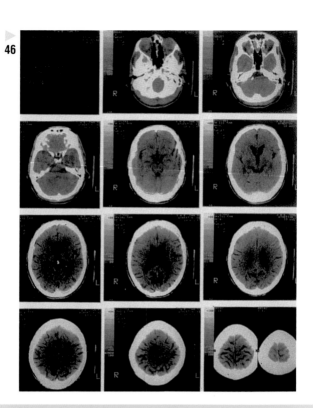

46 ▶ A 30-year-old man was arrested by the police for assaultive behavior and was noted to be disoriented and ataxic. His mother noted a loss of intellectual ability during the last year and the recent onset of "shoulder shrugs and twitches." His father had died at age 48 years in a nursing home, where he had been wheelchair-bound and demented for a number of years. A CT scan was obtained.

a) The most likely diagnosis is:
   1) Metachromatic leukodystrophy   3) Huntington's chorea
   2) Neurofibromatosis   4) Sturge-Weber syndrome

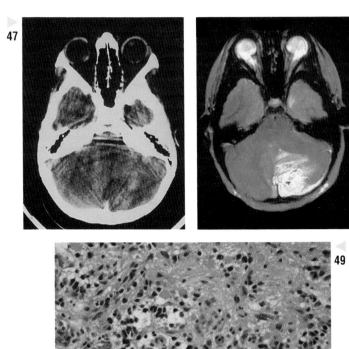

47-49 ▶ A 10-year-old boy had a 2-month history of headaches and gait ataxia. On the day of presentation, he had the sudden onset of a very severe headache and delirium. CT and MR scans are shown. A biopsy was performed. A photomicrograph of the biopsy shows hypercellularity and Rosenthal fibers.

a) What is the likely diagnosis?
   1) Hemorrhage into a preex-
      isting fibrocytic astrocy-
      toma of the cerebellum
   2) Meningioma
   3) Herpes simplex
      encephalitis
   4) Abscess

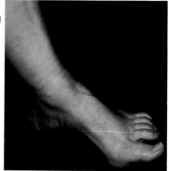

50 ▶ A 62-year-old woman had a lifelong history of bilateral ankle instability, mildly atrophic calf muscles, and thinning of the intrinsic muscles of the hands and feet. Nerve conduction studies demonstrated slowing of sensory and motor nerve conduction velocities.

a) Diagnosis, please.
b) There is a more severe form of this disease which affects infants and children. What is it?

51

	Right Carotid		
	Common	Internal	External
% Stenosis (diameter)	16-49	100	16-49
Plaque surface:			
Smooth	x	x	
Irregular			x
? Ulcerated			
Plaque composition:			
Homogeneous		x	x
Heterogeneous	x		

Peak velocity:	Right	Left	R EDV*	L EDV*
ICA	0	117	0	34
CCA	38	101		
ECA	101	85		

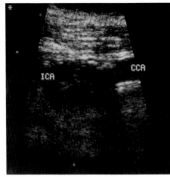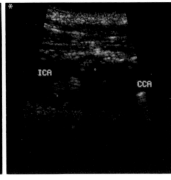

Left Carotid		
Common	Internal	External
16-49	16-49	16-49
x	x	
bulb x		x
x	x	
bulb x		

51-52 ▶ A 73-year-old man was noted by his wife to have new left lower facial weakness, which resolved in 16 hours. Noninvasive carotid imaging (NICI) study results are shown.

a) What do the NICIs show?
b) What therapeutic intervention should be taken?

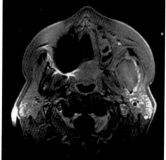

53 ▶ A 52-year-old woman complained of severe, lancinating left facial pain and evidenced xerostomia and trismus of the left musculus masseter on examination. Twenty years previously, squamous cell carcinoma of the frenulum of the tongue had been treated with 3000R by iridium implants and 4500R by external radiation.

a) What possible diagnoses might explain her pain?
b) What does the MR scan show?

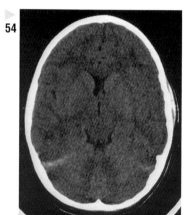

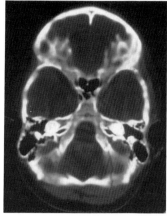

54-55 ▶ A 27-year-old woman slipped on the ice and struck her forehead on the pavement. She was briefly unconscious. Immediately thereafter she had a normal neurologic examination, but had hemotympanum on the left. CT scans without contrast and at the bone window setting are shown.

a) What are her diagnoses?

California Verbal Learning Test
  Recall   SS=46   (Mean=50, SD=10)
  Recognition   SS=-2   (Mean=0, SD=1)

Benton Visual Retention Test
  Correct   5
  Recognition   10

Trail Making Test
  Part A   34 seconds   percentile=25-50th
  Part B   51 seconds   percentile=75-90th

Purdue Pegboard Test
  Right 11   Left 10   Both 10

Halstead-Reitan Finger Tapping Test
  Right 33   Left 35

Benton Verbal Fluency Test
  RS=39   percentile=70-74th

Reading Sample (from Wide Range Achievement Test)
  SS=98   Grade level=13.0

Boston Naming Test
  RS=57

Mesulam Cancellation Test
  Nonverbal   Time 2'13"   omissions: Left 0   Right 0
  Verbal   Time 3'08"   omissions: Left 0   Right 1
  Nonverbal   Time 2'09"   omissions: Left 0   Right 0
  Verbal   Time 2'28"   omissions: Left 0   Right 0

Wisconsin Card Sort
  4 categories in 127 trials

---

56 ▶ A 36-year-old man was not wearing a helmet when he catapulted over the handlebars of his motorcycle, striking the left frontal area of his head on an oncoming vehicle. Thereafter, he had left frontal headache, lack of motivation, poor concentration, dizziness, and mood swings. CT and MR scans, EEGs including nasopharyngeal recordings and sleep deprivation, and a 24-hour ambulatory EEG were normal. Neuropsychologic test results are shown.

a) What diagnosis does the history suggest?

b) Does the neuropsychologic testing corroborate this diagnosis?

57-58 ▶ A 42-year-old malpractice attorney became intoxicated and took acquaintances for a 2-AM joyride in his Jaguar convertible. Shortly thereafter he failed to negotiate a turn and inverted his car in a stream. Rescuers took him to the hospital where he complained of neck pain and multiple bumps and bruises. Plain films of the cervical spine were interpreted as normal. He was kept for observation overnight, wearing a neck brace. The following dawn he had sobered up and was complaining of left shoulder pain extending into the biceps, accompanied by paresthesias in the left index finger and thumb. Examination revealed a slight weakness of the left biceps brachii, loss of left biceps and brachioradialis reflexes, and loss of pinprick sensation in the left index finger and thumb.

a) What is the differential diagnosis at this point?

case continues

▼

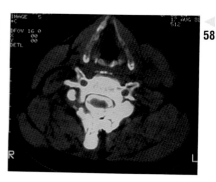

57

58

While being examined by the neurologist, the patient had transient symptoms of circumoral numbness, divergent gaze with horizontal diplopia, roaring tinnitus, right facial paresis, and left homonymous hemianopia.

b) What do these symptoms suggest and are they related to his neck injury?

c) What test would you choose to delineate the cause of these symptoms?

d) What do these images show?

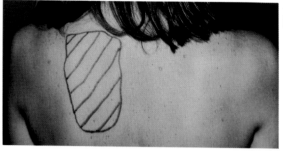

59 ▶ This 43-year-old assembly worker developed insidious onset of burning discomfort and numbness in the upper back as shown. MR scans of the cervical and thoracic spines were normal, as was the rest of the neurologic exam.

a) The most likely diagnosis is:

1) Diabetic neuropathy
2) Lung cancer metastatic to the scapula
3) Notalgia paresthetica
4) Neuralgic amyotrophy

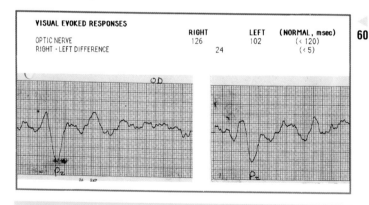

60 ▶ These visual evoked responses were obtained after the patient, a 49-year-old, otherwise healthy medical secretary, complained of her first episode of painful monocular visual loss in the left eye.

a) Diagnosis, please.

b) True or False: Oral adrenocorticosteroid therapy is indicated.

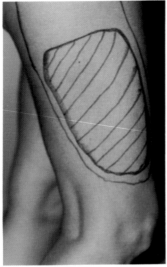

61 ▶ A 32-year-old woman attempted suicide by sedative overdose and was found unconscious in a squatting position in a hospital closet. After recovering from the overdose, she complained of pain and numbness in the distribution shown. Deep tendon reflexes were normal and there was no muscle weakness.

a) The most likely diagnosis is:
  1) Diabetic amyotrophy
  2) Aseptic necrosis of the femoral head
  3) Meralgia paraesthetica
  4) Herniated disc at L5-S1

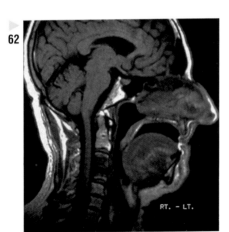

62 ▶ A 69-year-old man with no gag reflex aspirated during a modified barium swallow examination. An MR scan was obtained.

a) What does the MR scan reveal?
b) What is the most likely cause of failure of the gag reflex in this case?

63-64 ▶ This 12-year-old girl has metachromatic leukodystrophy. She weighs only 36 pounds and has profound weakness and intellectual deterioration. An EEG was obtained.

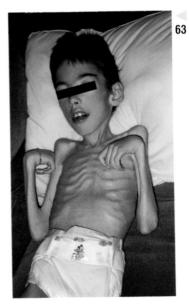

a) Which of the following is true?
1) This is a disease of the white matter.
2) Ataxia and hypotonia are usually followed by spasticity, amaurosis, and retinal degeneration.
3) White matter diseases are less likely than grey matter diseases to result in epilepsy.
4) All of the above.

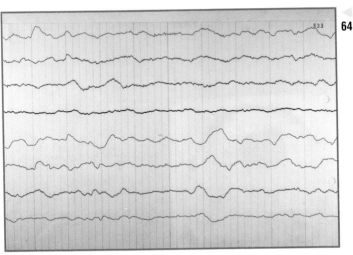

Olfactory Testing
University of Pennsylvania Smell Identification Test

UPSIT Score:	29	
	00-05	Nonphysiologic
	06-19	Anosmia
	20-33	Microsmia (Males)
	20-34	Microsmia (Females)
Normal:	34-40	Normosmia (Males)
Normal:	35-40	Normosmia (Females)

Impression: Microsmia

65 ▶ A 55-year-old woman who recently lost 110 pounds through dieting reported diminished smell and taste, without other signs or symptoms. Examination showed good ability to discriminate sweet, sour, bitter, and salty. The University of Pennsylvania Smell Identification Test score is shown. ENT evaluation; EEG; CT scan; and B_{12}, folic acid, and fasting glucose levels were within normal limits.

a) What contributes to a differential diagnosis of anosmia?

b) What is the most likely cause of the microsmia in this patient?

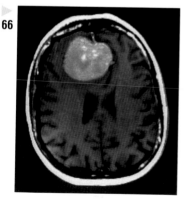

66 ▶ A 54-year-old woman with a normal neurologic examination volunteered for a study of age-associated memory impairment and had a screening MR scan.

a) What is the most likely diagnosis?
   1) Hemorrhagic infarction
   2) Giant aneurysm
   3) Meningioma of the falx cerebri
   4) Astrocytoma

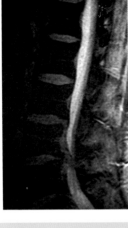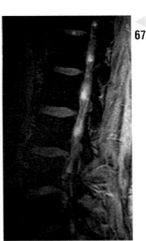

67 ▶ A 40-year-old man had received a medical discharge from the military for back pain several years prior. On presentation, he complained of back pain radiating into both lower extremities with greater pain into the right lower extremity. Valsalva maneuver increased the pain dramatically. An MR scan was obtained.

a) What does the MR scan show?

68 ▶ A 55-year-old woman was observed to have multiple episodes of left arm flexion and head deviation to the right lasting 5 to 10 seconds each. Episodic weakness of the left arm and leg had occurred over the previous 2 weeks. CT scan was normal. Eight days later, left hemiplegia, hemihypesthesia, hemianopsia, and right gaze preference occurred. An MR scan was obtained.

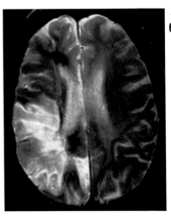

a) What does the MR scan reveal?

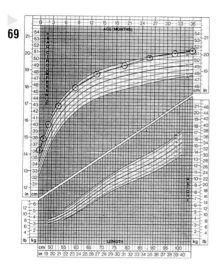

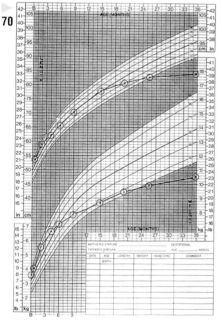

69-71 ▶ A 3-year-old girl was referred for gait disturbance and possible proximal muscle weakness. She was a child of professional parents and had received excellent prenatal care. Gestation and birth history were unremarkable. Birth weight was 8 pounds 12 ounces and her Apgar scores were 8 and 10 at 1 and 5 minutes, respectively. Growth initially was normal, but by the third year weight and height were beginning to fall off the curves (as shown) while head circumference remained normal.

a) In this case there is a disparity between head circumference (which is normal) and height/weight (which are low). Name several causes of macrocephaly.

case continues

▼

Motor skills in the first 1½ years were acquired on time, but she became unable to hop or climb stairs without pushing on her knee with one hand to stabilize herself (modified Gowers' sign). Gait was "waddling" in character, whether walking or running. She tended to become fatigued after just a few minutes of exertion, and would stop to rest. Her balance seemed fine, but she was easily knocked off her feet.

b) What is the general significance of proximal (hip and shoulder girdle) weakness, Gowers' sign, and a "waddling" gait?

case continues

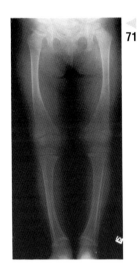

On examination she was noted to be a bright, happy child with a good attention span. She was quite dextrous. She had very mild weakness and easy fatigability in hip girdle and shoulder girdle muscles, as well as very slight bowing of the legs.

c) What diseases cause tibial bowing in combination with short stature?

case continues

On review of her family history, about half of the maternal relatives were noted to have relatively short stature, and several male relatives also had bowed legs and delayed walking in childhood. Laboratory work included normal ESR, CK, aldolase, glucose, and thyroid function tests. Serum calcium was normal, serum phosphate was low, and urine phosphate was elevated.

d) What familial disorder is the cause of this child's symptoms?

e) How is the condition treated, and what are the complications?

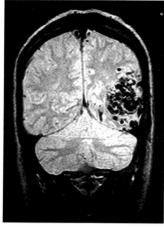

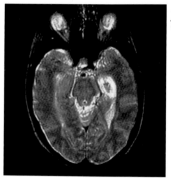

73 ► A 74-year-old man had a fever and mild delirium with loss of memory and sense of smell. A CT scan was normal. An MR scan taken 4 days after onset of illness is shown. CSF was remarkable for a lymphocytic pleocytosis, elevated protein, and a few RBCs with xanthochromia.

72 ► Recurrent left hemicranial throbbing headaches associated with scintillating scotomata, nausea, and vomiting plagued a 44-year-old man for 15 years. The headaches never generalized or occurred on the right side. Occasionally, he experienced paresthesias, weakness, and clumsiness in his right arm, and once his right arm and face twitched repeatedly for 10 minutes, during which time he could not speak.

a) What does the MR scan reveal?

b) What are the indications for surgery?

c) This lesion may present with:
   1) Seizures
   2) Migraine
   3) Subarachnoid hemorrhage
   4) All of the above

a) The most likely diagnosis is:
   1) Tuberculosis meningitis
   2) Stroke
   3) Encephalitis
   4) Bacterial meningitis

b) When this condition is suspected, which of the following is true?
   1) Acyclovir should be administered on an empiric basis.
   2) Acyclovir should never be administered without a diagnostic brain biopsy.
   3) An MR scan is more sensitive than a CT scan.

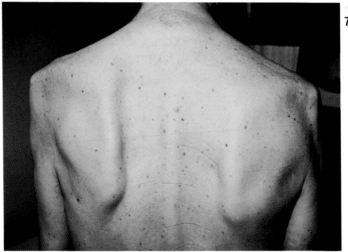

74-76 ▶ Slowly progressive paraplegia developed over 2 years in a 68-year-old man and was followed by weakness in the arms and neck flexors.

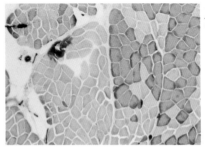

a) The most likely diagnosis is:
   1) Polymyositis
   2) Motor neuron disease (amyotrophic lateral sclerosis)
   3) Guillain-Barré syndrome
   4) Poliomyelitis
b) What features from the muscle biopsy indicate the pathologic diagnosis?

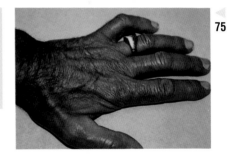

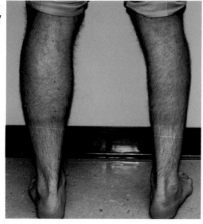

77 ▶ A 25-year-old man had weakness and atrophy of the right gastrocnemius muscle which developed over 8 years. All other muscles in his four limbs were normal. His CT-myelogram of the lumbosacral spine, CT scan of the pelvis, and neurologic exam were normal otherwise.

a) What would electromyography reveal?

b) Diagnosis, please.

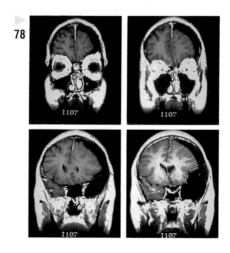

78 ▶ A 44-year-old fireman fell rounding third base at the annual fireman's picnic and softball game, striking his head lightly on the ground. A persistent headache mandated the CT scan shown, despite a normal neurologic examination.

a) Diagnosis, please.

79-80 ▶ A 70-year-old man had COPD and chronic atrial fibrillation, for which he was treated with coumadin. He complained of headache on awakening for 3 consecutive days and lightheadedness for 2 weeks. He had no ataxia, nausea, vomiting, true vertigo, or diplopia. Poor right foot tapping and a tendency to lean to the right on testing tandem gait were noted. MR (79) and CT (80) scans were obtained.

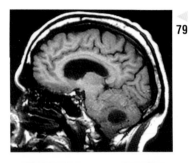

79

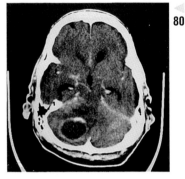

80

a) What does the MR scan reveal?
b) What secondary complications might occur with this lesion?

81 ▶ The patient described in the previous case was doing well after removal of his astrocytoma until 9 months later when he suddenly developed weakness of the left face and arm, which resolved over 7 hours. A CT scan was obtained.

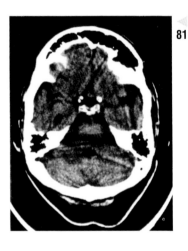

81

a) Does the CT scan indicate a recurrence of tumor?
b) What is the most likely diagnosis?
c) What other diagnostic studies should be performed?

82

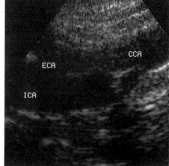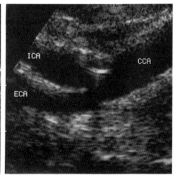

83

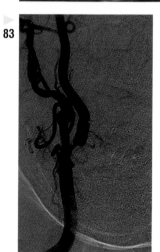

82-83 ▶ A 62-year-old woman reported total loss of vision in her right eye for 5 minutes approximately 1 week prior. A loud right carotid bruit was auscultated.

a) What do the noninvasive carotid imaging studies and the digital subtraction angiogram show?
b) What is the recommended treatment?

84 ▶ A 40-year-old physician noted fasciculations in his left gastrocnemius muscle. Over 3 years, they were noted sporadically in the other leg, buttocks, chest wall anteriorly and posteriorly, both arms, and even the neck. While worse after exercise, drinking coffee, or when fatigued, they never affected the tongue or face. No weakness or reflex change was detectable on examination.

a) Where do fasciculations originate?
b) Are fasciculations ever benign?
c) What tests might be considered at this point?

85 ▶ A 71-year-old man was brought in for treatment by a family member because of slowly progressive memory loss and two recent automobile accidents. The patient denied problems, although impaired attention, orientation, concentration, and short-term memory characterized his otherwise-normal examination. CT scan, EEG, B_{12}, folate, VDRL, and thyroid function studies were normal. Despite being instructed not to drive, the following month he was observed driving down the road apparently unaware of flames coming from beneath his car, which thereupon exploded, killing him.

According to Vernon Police an eyewitness saw ■■■■ car on fire traveling east on Newton Road. Moments later it was engulfed in flames.

Another eyewitness, ■■■■ ■■■■ of Vernon, said she was at the intersection of Governor Hunt Road and Route 142 between 7:30 and 7:40 a.m., and saw a blue car heading in the opposite direction with flames and sparks coming from the back driver's side tire. She said there was a very strong smell of rubber.

"The smell was so bad, I don't know how he couldn't have noticed it," she said.

a) What is the most likely diagnosis?

b) How can you account for the fact that he did not appear to notice the smell of burning rubber?

86 ▶ A 63-year-old woman had a whiplash injury. On examination in the emergency room she was noted to have atrophy of the intrinsic hand muscles, numbness over both shoulders, and hyperreflexia in the lower extremities. Her MR scan is shown.

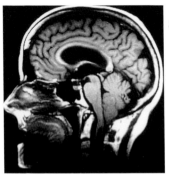

a) Diagnosis, please.

b) Is this a result of her accident?

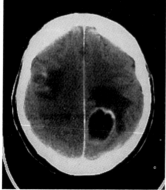

Verbal IQ = 119
Performance IQ = 121
Full scale IQ = 120

Wechsler Memory Scale Score

132

87 ▸ A 67-year-old man status post resection of small cell carcinoma of the lung presented with a several-day history of right leg weakness and a 4-week history of acalculia, memory loss, and labile affect. A CT scan of his brain was obtained.

88 ▸ A 78-year-old woman complained of forgetfulness, a tendency to get lost while driving, lack of initiative, anorexia, and excessive sleepiness. Her neurologic examination was normal and her Mini–Mental State score was 29 of 30. Her Wechsler Adult Intelligence Scale–Revised and Wechsler Memory Scale scores are shown.

a) Which of the following statements is true of brain metastasis?

1) Affected individuals usually die of the brain metastasis rather than the primary tumor.
2) Mental status change is an unusual presenting symptom of brain metastasis.
3) Overall morbidity is improved by resection of a solitary metastasis.
4) The potential risks of dexamethasone outweigh its benefits in treating patients with brain metastasis.

a) This patient has:

1) Dementia of the Alzheimer type
2) Metabolic encephalopathy
3) Pseudodementia
4) Hysteria

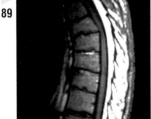
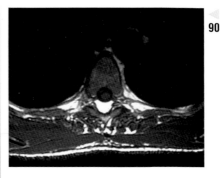

89-90 ► A 43-year-old man who had been treated with steroids for several years had within the prior few weeks noted painless bilateral leg weakness with flexor spasms of the legs during the night. On examination he had a mild spastic paraparesis, with bilateral ankle clonus and extensor plantar responses. Thoracic MR scan is shown in sagittal and axial planes.

a) What is the diagnosis?

91 ► A dense left hemiplegia occurred suddenly in a 47-year-old man who had no known risk factors for stroke. A carotid angiogram was obtained.

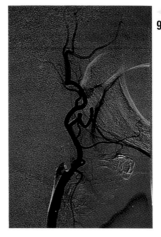

a) What does the angiogram show?
b) What are the risk factors for this lesion?

92-95 ▶ An 83-year-old woman with hypertension, degenerative joint disease, and iron-deficiency anemia was admitted for progressive right leg weakness. General slowing of motor abilities had caused her to rely on a walker for the previous 2 years. She had fallen 2 weeks prior, without injury. No tremor, drooling, bradykinesia, or stiffness were reported, and she also denied prior stroke, transient ischemic attack, head trauma, loss of consciousness, or incontinence. On exam, she was anxious and tremulous, cooperating only after repeated commands. Marked paratonia without cogwheel rigidity, mild right hemiparesis, and dystaxic finger-nose-finger were found. Her gait was wide-based and "magnetic," especially on the right, but all other neurologic signs were normal. Reflexes were hyperactive throughout and plantar signs were extensor bilaterally. A small nontender, nonfixed nodule was noted above the left inner canthus of the eye.

a) What conditions might present in this manner?

b) What test(s) would you order first?

case continues

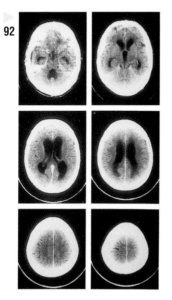

92

A CT scan of the brain is shown.

c) Are there findings of significance on the CT scan?

case continues

As the facial nodule was new, it was biopsied and revealed mature squamous epithelium with infiltrative chronic inflammatory cells and clear capsules containing round, gray inclusion bodies thought to be *Cryptococcus*.

d) What test would you recommend next?

case continues

Results for this test are shown in the accompanying table.

e) What are the typical cerebrospinal fluid (CSF) findings in chronic meningitis?

f) Is this a case of "normal pressure hydrocephalus"?

case continues

Opening pressure (mmCSF)	160	**93**
RBC (per HPF)	20	
WBC (per HPF)	11	
Differential:		
%Neutrophils	0	
%Mononuclear cells	100	
Total protein (mg%)	218	
Glucose (mg%)	19	
Gram's stain	negative	
Bacterial culture	negative	
Cytology	negative	
India ink prep	positive	
Cryptococcal antigen	positive	

94

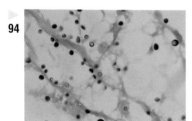

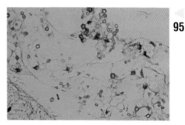

95

Despite intravenous amphotericin B and oral flucytosine, repeat lumbar punctures continued to demonstrate cryptococcal organisms. Renal failure set in after 6 weeks of therapy, and the patient died. Sections of the meninges are shown.

g) Does cryptococcal meningitis occur only in immunosuppressed hosts?

T$_3$ Uptake	27.4
T$_4$	8.3
FT$_1$	2.3
RPR	nonreactive
B$_{12}$	293
ESR	4
Ethanol	none detected
CT head	normal
EEG	normal

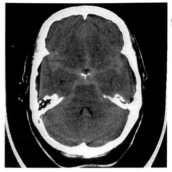

96 ▶ A 58-year-old high school vocational counselor was asked by the high school principal to seek medical advice for a "personality change." Neurologic examination, Mini–Mental State score, CT, EEG, B$_{12}$, folate, thyroid function studies, and VDRL were all normal. Six months later, his paranoia and forgetfulness resulted in admission to a mental health unit. Diffuse cerebral dysfunction was found on formal neuropsychologic testing. Signs now included disinhibited snout, glabellar blink, and nuchocephalic reflexes along with impairment of upward gaze and paratonia in the limbs.

a) What is the most likely diagnosis?

97 ▶ A 29-year-old aerobics instructor in excellent health experienced the sudden onset of the "worst headache of [her] life." A neurologic examination was completely normal. Her CT scan (without contrast) is shown.

a) Diagnosis, please.
b) Which of the following is true?
   1) A CT scan can show up to 85% of subarachnoid hemorrhages within the first 24 hours and may eliminate the need for a cerebrospinal fluid examination by lumbar puncture.
   2) In this era, more than 90% of persons with subarachnoid hemorrhage will have an excellent recovery.
   3) If no aneurysm is seen on an MR scan, there is really no need to perform cerebral angiography.
   4) Trauma is a more common cause of subarachnoid hemorrhage than is aneurysmal rupture.

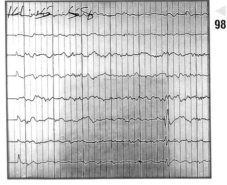

98 ▶ This EEG segment is from a 24-hour ambulatory recording in a 55-year-old man with recurrent episodes of unresponsiveness, during one of which his car left the road and rolled twice while he was driving. On another occasion, he was found on the floor in a crouched position, groveling and grunting. He had no recall of any of the events.

a) What is the electroencephalographic finding?

b) What is the treatment of choice?

99 ▶ This 68-year-old woman had a lacunar stroke in the right hemisphere 1 year previously, with resolution since then. Recently she presented with bilateral eyelid ptosis, worse on the left. With her eyelids held open, she had a third-nerve palsy of eye movements on the left only. CT scans of the head and chest were normal. Acetylcholine receptor antibodies were slightly elevated.

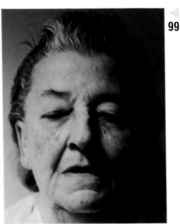

a) Diagnosis, please.
b) What diagnostic test is likely to prove useful?

100 ▶ A 52-year-old man with a 20-year history of migraine headaches suffered the acute onset of the "worst headache of [his] life" while having sexual intercourse.

a) Is coital cephalgia more likely to be due to a benign or a malignant cause?

case continues

Although this patient has had prior headaches, the current presentation represented a dramatic change in pattern in that no prior episode had been so severe, so sudden in onset, or associated with exertion.

b) What is the most ominous diagnosis that should be considered?

case continues

The neurologic examination was entirely normal. There was no meningism, and Kernig's and Brudzinski's signs were absent.

c) Should any diagnostic tests be done?

case continues

100

RBC (per HPF)	7000	3000
WBC (per HPF)	100 (100% lymphs)	42 (100% lymphs)
Total protein (mg%)	40	
Glucose (mg%—serum glucose 100)	67	
Xanthochromia	None	None

Opening pressure: 180 mmCSF
Closing pressure: 170 mmCSF

A CT scan was normal. The results of cerebrospinal fluid examination 2 hours after onset of the headache are shown.

d) Are these data more consistent with a traumatic tap or with subarachnoid hemorrhage?

case continues

Given all the data, there was a complete discussion of alternatives with the patient.

e) Should this event now be considered a variant of migraine or should an angiogram be done to further investigate the problem?

case ends

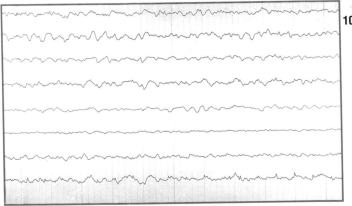

101

101-102 ▶ This EEG was obtained while a 52-year-old woman had intermittent twitching in the right arm for over 1 hour. Unresponsiveness with head deviation to the left alternated with brief intervals of semipurposeful right arm movements to command.

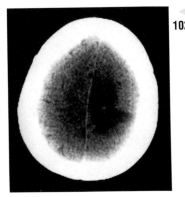

102

a) Diagnosis, please.
b) What does the CT scan demonstrate?

103

Opening pressure	170 mmCSF
WBC (per HPF)	5
RBC (per HPF)	0
Total protein (mg%)	57
Oligoclonal bands	present

103 ▶ A 34-year-old man presented with axial and appendicular ataxia. Over 48 hours, horizontal gaze failed and the next day his extraocular muscles were totally paralyzed. Within a week, pain in the shoulders emerged, accompanied by weakness in serratus anterior, biceps, and deltoid muscles, bilaterally, worse on the right. All reflexes were absent. Cerebrospinal fluid analysis is shown.

a) Diagnosis, please.

b) What most likely explains the shoulder pain and shoulder-girdle muscle weakness?

104

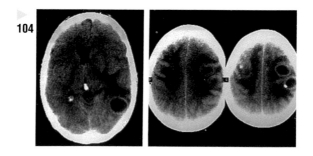

104 ▶ A 52-year-old man with a history of alcohol abuse had a nagging upper respiratory infection and presented with mental status change, a temperature of 101.6°F, and bilateral upper extremity weakness. His CT scan is shown.

a) Which of the following are likely?

1) The lesions are probably abscesses.
2) Alcohol abuse is a risk factor.
3) Similar ring-enhancing lesions can occur in metastatic cancer.
4) Stereotaxic biopsy is indicated.
5) All of the above.

105 ▶ A 60-year-old airline pilot noticed during his last several flights that when he extended his neck to check overhead instruments he predictably developed diplopia followed by complete loss of vision in both eyes. Symptoms resolved within seconds after he repositioned his neck. An MR angiogram was obtained.

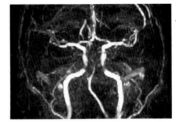

a) What does the angiogram show?
b) Should he continue his career?

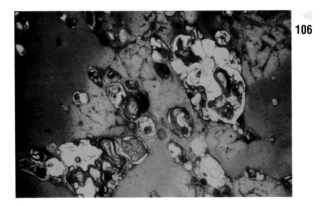

106 ▶ A 58-year-old campground operator slowly developed bilateral footdrop over 2 years. While reflexes were diminished in general, there was no sensory loss, ataxia, or sphincter disturbance. Fasciculations were absent. A left gastrocnemius muscle biopsy revealed rimmed vacuoles, which were examined under an electron microscope (shown above).

a) Diagnosis, please.
b) What would you expect electromyography to reveal?
c) True or False: Adrenocorticosteroid therapy helps patients with this disease.

107 ▶ A 71-year-old man with a long history of alcoholism had, several months prior, reduced his intake to 6 to 8 ounces of whiskey each day. The day after a Thanksgiving feast, he developed an acute change in mental status. All tests, including metabolic screen for delirium and thyroid function, liver enzyme, vitamin B_{12}, and folic acid studies, were normal.

a) What would be the value of checking serum ammonia or CSF glutamine in this context?

case continues

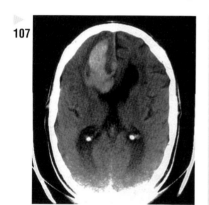

107

The serum ammonia was normal; CSF examination was deferred. When the neurologist examined the patient, she noted that he was oriented fully and scored 30/30 on the Mini–Mental State Examination. He was extremely apathetic, indolent, and slow-moving, all of which were new characteristics according to the family. A CT scan was recommended and is shown.

b) How could this be explained?

case continues

The following day, while eating breakfast, the patient suddenly began to stare, then cried out, raised his left arm, turned his head and eyes as if to look at his left hand, and maintained this posture for 2 minutes. He then resumed eating.

c) What was this event?

108 ▶ An old man, according to a family member, "bumped his head, went to bed, and didn't get up in the morning." His CT scan is shown.

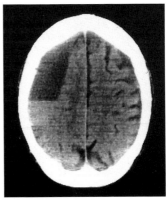

a) Diagnosis, please.
b) What are some of the CT characteristics that contribute to such a diagnosis?

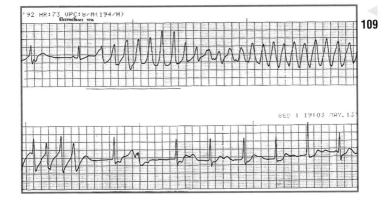

109 ▶ A 69-year-old woman had several episodes of syncope with several hours of confusion as an aftermath. The events were not witnessed at onset. A cardiac monitor verified the disturbance shown.

a) These events were probably due to:
   1) Ventricular fibrillation due to status epilepticus
   2) Neurocardiac reflex secondary to subarachnoid hemorrhage
   3) Torsade de pointes secondary to quinidine
   4) Epilepsia partialis continua

Muscle	Insertional Activity	Fibrillations	Positive Sharp Waves
R ADM	Normal	0	0
R APB	Normal	0	0
R 1st DI	Normal	0	0
R Biceps	Increased	0	0
*R Deltoid	Increased	0	0
*R Triceps	Increased	0	0
*R Tibialis ant	Increased	0	0
*R Gastroc/sol	Increased	0	0
*R Vastus med	Increased	0	0
R Paraspinous	Normal	0	0

*Evidence low-amplitiude highly polyphasic potentials with increased recruitment at submaximal firing rates.

110-111 ▶ A 6-year-old boy bumped his left shin and complained of local pain. Thereafter, he was noted to have trouble walking over uneven ground, to pull himself upstairs by using his arms on the bannister rail, and to be unable to get up off the floor by himself. He denied sensory complaints and bowel or bladder dysfunction. Examination revealed 4/5 neck flexor, bilateral biceps, triceps, hip flexor, hamstring, and foot dorsiflexor functions. Gowers' sign was positive. Sensation and reflexes were normal. Plantar signs were flexor. The CK was 552 IU/L (normal = 85-232 IU/L). Electromyographic (EMG) studies were obtained.

a) This EMG report is most consistent with:
1) Neuropathy
2) Neuromuscular transmission defect
3) Myopathy
4) Fibromyalgia

b) What would you do next?
1) Start steroid treatment and obtain a right quadriceps muscle biopsy
2) Obtain a left quadriceps muscle biopsy and then start steroid treatment
3) Start steroid treatment and obtain a left quadriceps muscle biopsy
4) Obtain a right quadriceps muscle biopsy and then start steroid treatment

Fasciculations	Firing Rate	Interference Pattern	Amplitude (max mV)
0	High	Full	5
0	High	Full	4
0	High	Full	5
0	High	Full	2
0	High	Full	1
0	High	Full	1
0	High	Full	2
0	High	Full	2
0	High	Full	3
0	High	Full	5

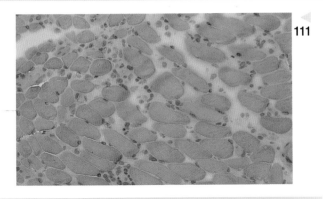

111

With prednisone 40 mg/d, dramatic clinical improvement was accompanied by a fall in the CK to 510 IU/L in less than a week, at which time a left quadriceps (to avoid the confusion induced by needle EMG in the right leg) muscle biopsy was obtained (shown). Prednisone was decreased to 30 mg/d; however, within a week he had deteriorated and was weaker than noted initially. The steroid dose was increased to 40 mg/d with slow recovery over 3 weeks. The CK fell to 210 IU/L.

c) What is the diagnosis?

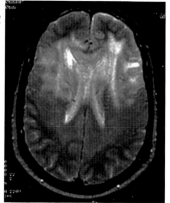

112 ► A 56-year-old bank executive who had subacute loss of cognitive function had a normal neurologic examination, except for extreme apathy and bradykinesia.

a) From the MR scan, the likely diagnostic possibilities include:
1) "Butterfly" glioblastoma of the corpus callosum and both frontal lobes
2) Primary histiocytic lymphoma of the CNS
3) Adrenoleukodystrophy
4) All of the above

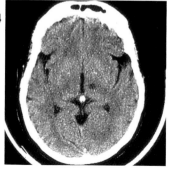

113 ► A 76-year-old woman complained of diplopia and increasing difficulty walking over several months. On examination she had facial diparesis and dysarthria with appendicular and truncal ataxia. CT scan and lumbar puncture were normal. An MR scan was obtained.

a) Diagnosis, please.

114 ►

a) This patient's CT scan most likely represents a thalamic:
1) Hemorrhagic infarct
2) Plaque of demyelination
3) Tumor
4) Stereotactic radio-frequency lesion for intractable benign essential tremor

115-116 ▶ A 62-year-old, right-handed woman with the recent onset of unexplained headaches reported having had "brain fever" at the age of 9 years. Birth and developmental history were otherwise normal as was her current neurologic examination. A CT scan and an EEG were obtained.

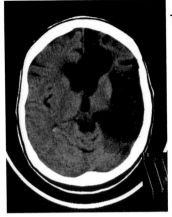

115

a) What do the patient's CT scan and EEG reveal?

116

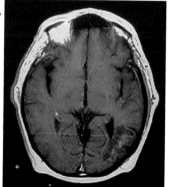

117 ▶ A 50-year-old woman with an inability to concentrate while reading and intermittent right-hand paresthesias had extinction of visual and somatosensory stimulation on the right. An MR scan was obtained.

a) What does the MR scan reveal?
b) What other signs might be found on examination?

118

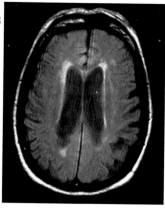

118 ▶ A 75-year-old woman was noted by her husband to have poor memory, frequent falls, and incontinence. An MR scan was obtained.

a) What is seen on her MR scan?
b) What test would you order next?

119 **University of Pennsylvania Smell Identification Test (UPSIT) Score:**

3 Correct (of a possible 40)

119 ▶

a) This is most consistent with:
  1) Malingering
  2) Olfactory groove meningioma
  3) Mild parkinsonism
  4) A history of closed head trauma

120 ► A 45-year-old man complained of multiple episodes of true vertigo without a positional component over the previous 3 weeks. Twenty-five years prior to the episodic vertigo, transient unilateral tinnitus and dulling of vision in the right eye lasted for 2 days. Neurologic exam was normal. An MR scan was obtained.

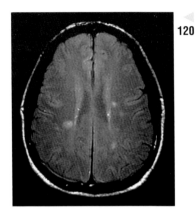

a) What are the possible diagnoses?
b) What are the findings on the MR scan?

121 ► On routine eye examination, a 23-year-old woman was incidentally noted to have downbeat nystagmus (rapid phase down) in both eyes in primary position and on lateral gaze in either direction. MR imaging of her head was performed.

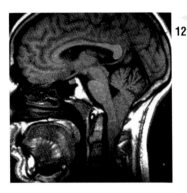

a) The most likely cause of this nystagmus in her case is:
   1) Meningioma of foramen magnum
   2) Phenytoin overdose
   3) Chiari malformation
   4) Demyelinating disease
   5) Remote effect of carcinoma
   6) Lithium toxicity

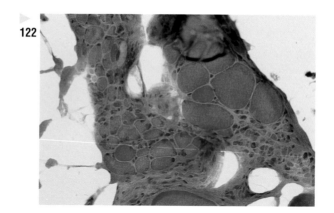

122

122 ▶ Over 18 months, a 78-year-old woman with mild non–insulin-dependent diabetes mellitus developed weakness, inability to walk, and aching of the shoulders and hips. Arising from a seated position was difficult, requiring assistance or walking of her hands up her thighs (Gowers' sign). Electromyography demonstrated low-amplitude, polyphasic potentials with increased recruitment on submaximal voluntary contraction of proximal arm and leg muscles. Scattered fibrillations and positive sharp waves were also found, but fasciculations were absent. A left biceps muscle biopsy is shown.

a) Diagnosis, please.

b) Why do signs of neurogenic denervation occur in this condition?

123-126 ▶ A 33-year-old woman developed behavior changes over 1 year. These consisted of apathy alternating with intervals of agitation, mania, and depression. She had been treated with modest success with lithium, allowing her to carry on as a bookkeeper until she developed polydipsia and polyuria and began acting violently toward animate and inanimate objects alike. At one point she put her cat in the freezer.

a) What intracranial lesion might produce these symptoms?

case continues

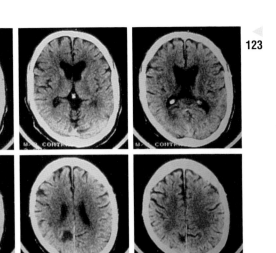

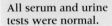

All serum and urine
tests were normal.

b) CT scan of the brain
was obtained and
shows:
1) Hydrocephalus
2) Agenesis of the
corpus callosum
3) Frontotemporal
atrophy
4) Demyelinating
disease
c) The EEG reveals:
1) Mild bifrontal
slowing
2) Epileptiform
discharges
3) Sleep spindles
4) Normal rhythms

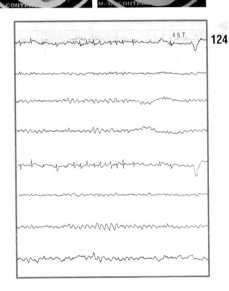

case continues

case continues

125

Opening pressure (mmCSF)	80	Fungal culture	negative
RBC (per HPF)	0	Bacterial culture	negative
WBC (per HPF)	0	AFB culture	negative
Differential:		India ink prep	negative
%Neutrophils	0	Cryptococcal antigen	negative
%Mononuclear cells	0	Myelin basic protein	negative
Total protein (mg%)	34	Gamma globulin fraction	9%
Glucose (mg%)	79	Oligoclonal bands	negative
Glutamine	0	Cytology	negative
Gram's stain	negative	VDRL	negative

Cerebrospinal fluid analysis is shown in the accompanying table. Her condition deteriorated over 6 months to the point where she was unconcerned about household chores, holidays, or family matters. Judgment and insight were severely impaired but, nonetheless, her memory, calculation and language functions remained quite good. Examination was remarkable for akathisia, perseverations, motor impersistence, and disinhibited snout and bilateral palmomental reflexes. In this previously healthy young person with an 18-month history of cognitive and behavioral decline, a brain biopsy was obtained from the right frontal lobe. It revealed nonspecific gliosis and some neuronal dropout without pathognomonic changes of any known neurodegenerative or infectious disorder.

d) Possible diagnoses include:
    1) AIDS–dementia complex
    2) Non-Alzheimer (lobar) dementia
    3) Pick's disease
    4) All of the above

case continues

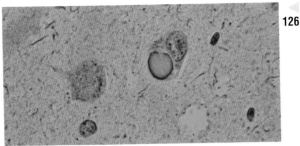

Because of financial constraints, the patient was subsequently cared for at home for several more months. Medications included lithium, 1200 mg/d; thioridazine, 150 mg/d; and amitriptyline, 200 mg/d. She was found dead at the kitchen table one afternoon just before her husband's birthday. Autopsy revealed a lethal amitriptyline level in the blood and the death was ruled a suicide.

e) What is the postmortem pathologic diagnosis shown in the figure?

case ends

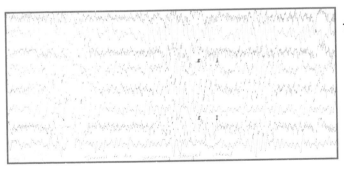

127 ▶ A 3-year-old girl with a family history of primary generalized epilepsy was seen for staring attacks and apparently intentional disobedience. An EEG was obtained.

a) What does the EEG show?

b) How does this case differ from typical absence epilepsy?

▶ Answers:

1 a) Hemangioblastoma, ependymoma, syringomyelia.

b) Treatment with carbamazepine, amitriptyline, or baclofen might reduce the unpleasant dysesthesias.

2 a) Cheiralgia paresthetica. This condition is caused by injury to the sensory branch of the radial nerve in the forearm and has been reported as a consequence of handcuffs.

3 a) Meningioma.

b) Carbamazepine. Ethosuximide is a first-line anticonvulsant for epilepsy (petit mal) in children. Clonazepam is a second-line adjuvant anticonvulsant used in conjunction with a first-line agent such as phenytoin or carbamazepine to control refractory epilepsy after monotherapy trials have failed.

c) Valproic acid. When used with clonazepam, this combination therapy may result in absence status epilepticus and is therefore strictly contraindicated.

4 a) Basilar impression of the brainstem. Chiari malformation is also seen. All of the patient's symptoms were reversed by an anterior odontoidectomy.

5 a) Spondylitic myelopathy. Cervical spondylosis is a common cause of mild-to-moderate stenosis of the spinal canal. The resultant spasticity may be "subclinical" in the elderly and contribute to a more generalized gait disturbance.

6 a) Absolutely yes. When the conventional cerebral angiogram was obtained, it showed a 12-mm posterior communicating artery aneurysm, which was successfully treated surgically.

7-8 a) Right middle cerebral artery anterior branch distribution hypodensity consistent with nonhemorrhagic stroke.

b) Embolism from chronic atrial fibrillation or, less likely, embolism from ulcerated plaque in the right internal carotid artery.

9 a) Tension headache, cervical spondylosis, and mass lesions at the foramen magnum.

b) An extradural defect at C1-2 thought to be either neoplasm or vascular anomaly. Despite normal angiography, surgical repair of an aberrant right vertebral artery compressing the C1 and C2 roots relieved the complaints.

10-11 a) The MR scan demonstrates a right posterior cerebral artery stroke. Absence of the right internal carotid artery and left vertebral artery is seen on the MR angiogram.

b) While status migraine must be considered, these symptoms most likely occurred on an ischemic basis.

c) Auditory musical hallucinations occur most commonly in the setting of otosclerosis, but may also signify lesions of the temporal lobe(s).

12-14 a) There is a mass lesion with rim enhancement within the left frontotemporal region. There is considerable midline shift and edema.

b) The acute deterioration in neurologic condition in the presence of fever suggests an infectious etiology, and the images suggest probable abscess formation. The CT scan also shows apparent direct extension of the tumor mass from the paranasal sinuses into the middle cranial fossa.

c) This is a case of "benign" nasal polyposis with eventual pressure erosion of the base of the skull, and invasion into the braincase. Note the presence of respiratory epithelium, without malignant change.

15-16 a) All of the above.

b) Acoustic neuroma.

17 a) Posttraumatic syringomyelia.

b) Lower extremity spasticity and weakness; upper extremity flaccidity, atrophy, and weakness; ataxia; and incontinence.

18 a) Progressive supranuclear palsy (Steele-Richardson-Olszewski syndrome).

b) Yes. Progressive cognitive decline accompanies many such cases even though the primary pathology (neuronal dropout and amyloid plaques) appears confined to the pretectal region of the brainstem leading some to distinguish this as a subcortical dementia in contrast to a dementia of the Alzheimer type, which derives primarily from loss of cortical and hippocampal dendritic synaptic boutons and neurons.

19 a) Internuclear ophthalmoplegia. This is due to involvement of the medial longitudinal fasciculus which links the nuclei of cranial nerves III, IV, and VI. It is often bilateral because of the proximity of these fasciculi to one another.

In an elderly person, vascular insufficiency is more likely the cause. In a young person, demyelinating disease should be suspected.

20 a) All are true. There are very characteristic physical features in the various mucopolysaccaridoses recognizable by simple inspection.

21 a) Complex partial seizure.

   b) Mesial temporal sclerosis versus low-grade glioma (note area of hyperintensity in the left temporal lobe).

22 a) Cervical myelopathy secondary to extradural compression.

   b) A large posterior osteophyte at C4-5 and a smaller one at C6-7, resulting in variable degrees of spinal stenosis.

23 a) The CT shows a large extradural defect at L5-S1 on the right.

   b) Not likely. The S1 nerve root is being distorted by the disc fragment. It is possible that conservative intervention would alleviate the pain; however, the pressure on the S1 nerve root would remain, which could lead to motor and sensory deficit.

24 a) A traumatic left occipital lobe contusion.

25 a) Apparent acute or subacute change in mental status could be due to toxic or metabolic encephalopathy (including drug overdose), traumatic injury to the brain, subarachnoid hemorrhage, brain tumor (sometimes with an irritative meningitis secondary to contents of ruptured tumor cyst), or complex partial status epilepticus (versus postictal state).

   b) All of these signs are consistent with normal wakefulness and embellishment, suggesting strongly an hysterical conversion reaction. Toxic-metabolic workup was negative.

   c) Additional support for the diagnosis derives from the EEG pattern shown. There is a normal background of posterior 10-11 Hertz alpha rhythm and anterior 15-25 Hertz beta rhythm. No epileptiform activity, asymmetry, or slowing were noted. While coma can occur in some cases showing diffuse alpha rhythms ("alpha coma"), the posterior predominant alpha in combination with beta activity anteriorly is really only consistent with normal wakefulness.

   d) Management is very challenging because no treatment has been effective in reversing conversion reactions directly. In general, it is best for all staff to provide a supportive, encouraging milieu without becoming confrontational or judgmental. Usually within a short time, embellishment is replaced by a cry for psychiatric help. The principal risk is that of suicide, since conversion reactions represent extremely low-level defense mechanisms.

26-28 a) Diabetic amyotrophy.

b) Diffuse diabetic sensorimotor polyneuropathy.

c) False.

d) False.

e) To rule out thymoma.

f) Posterior mediastinal adenopathy.

g) True.

h) Sarcoidosis.

i) No. Positive ARA titers are reported in patients with sarcoidosis and represent an epiphenomenon in the absence of abnormal clinical signs and neurophysiologic testing for myasthenia gravis.

j) No. The MR findings in patients with neurosarcoidosis, who often express oligoclonal bands in the CSF, consist of white matter hyperintensities similar in appearance to plaques of demyelination found in multiple sclerosis. These were originally thought to occur preferentially in the perihypothalamic area at the base of the brain; however, enlarging experience has shown that all of the cerebral white matter is susceptible to infiltration by sarcoid.

29 a) Atypical absence epilepsy characterized by recurrent diffuse spike and wave discharges. If these were occurring at a rate of 3/s, the symptoms would qualify for the diagnosis of petit mal epilepsy.

b) Ethosuximide and valproic acid. With other associated seizure manifestations (focal or generalized motor activity), valproic acid is the treatment of choice.

30 a) Pontine glioma. This is the most ominous of the infratentorial tumors in childhood, with a uniformly grave prognosis. Houndsfield unit artifact in CT scans makes visualization of the pons nearly impossible, but MR imaging clearly shows the tumor.

31 a) All of the above. Clinically, it was felt the patient had multiple sclerosis.

32 a) Lateral recess stenosis at L4-5 on the right, producing an L5 radiculopathy.

33 a) Large herniated disc at L5-S1 with compression of the right S1 root.

 b) Yes. CT or MR scans would probably have led to the diagnosis (and surgical correction), thus avoiding chronic pain, atrophy, and weakness.

34 a) Demyelinating disease. The patient has had both right hemisphere, left hemisphere, and dorsal column involvement disseminated in time and space. Vascular or neoplastic disease would be less likely explanations for a left hemiparesis at age 16 years.

 b) Multifocal white matter abnormalities, some of which enhance, consistent with demyelinating disease.

35-36 a) Fibrotic scar tissue. Although disc material can uncommonly enhance, this is most likely scar tissue. Lipomata are intensely white, even without enhancement, because of their high fat content.

37 a) A right parietal mass lesion with little edema, which pathologically was a grade I astrocytoma.

 b) Despite normal EEGs, these symptoms were thought most likely to be complex partial seizures. She responded to carbamazepine.

38-41 a) A myopathy, possibly a reversible side effect of lovastatin.

 b) No. Lovastatin-induced myopathy need not cause inflammatory muscle changes to appear in the serum (elevated CK and ESR).

 c) Multilevel acute denervation in all muscles sampled, most likely because of diffuse motor neuronopathy.

 d) Yes. It makes neuropathy more likely.

 e) If a muscle biopsy were needed, prior needle EMG testing would result in an "inflammatory" response throughout the needled muscle, leading to an incorrect diagnosis of polymyositis or at least obscuring the true diagnosis. As the left leg is in this category, sparing the contralateral limb for biopsy is appropriate.

 f) No. The neuropathy may, in fact, be primary motor neuron disease.

 g) A right gastrocnemius muscle biopsy.

 h) Although it is consistent with neuropathy, the muscle biopsy findings are nonspecific and do not reveal fiber-type grouping, which would point strongly toward ALS as the diagnosis. As it turned out, the mitochondria noted on electronmicroscopy were not identified as abnormal by enzymatic assay.

i) CT scans of the lumbosacral spine and pelvis to exclude nerve root compression intra- and extrathecally.

j) Familial ALS with incidental lumbar radiculopathy.

42-43 a) Internal carotid–middle cerebral artery aneurysm.

b) Carbamazepine. It has been reported to cause a dense metabolic encephalopathy resembling akinetic mutism or persistent vegetative state in patients after various forms of brain injury.

44 a) Cogan's syndrome.

b) Oral adrenocorticosteroid medication.

45 a) A neoplasm of the cervical spinal cord (ependymoma).

b) Multiple sclerosis and neoplasm.

46 a) Huntington's chorea. There is atrophy of the caudate nuclei bilaterally, although cerebral atrophy has not yet taken place.

47-49 a) Hemorrhage into an astrocytoma. In children, infratentorial tumors are more common than supratentorial tumors. In this instance, bleeding into the tumor resulted in an acute presentation and earlier detection. Total resection was achieved in this case. Complete surgical cure is usually possible with this tumor type.

50 a) Hereditary sensorimotor polyneuropathy type 1-demyelinating (HSMN-I, Charcot-Marie-Tooth syndrome).

b) HSMN-III (Dejerine-Sottas syndrome).

51-52 a) Large irregular plaque at the origin of the right internal carotid artery with an absent Doppler signal distal to the plaque, suggestive of total or near total occlusion, and moderate stenosis in the left internal carotid artery. Angiography confirmed complete obstruction of the right internal carotid artery.

b) Since the patient has complete occlusion of the affected side, no further action need be taken at present. He should be scheduled for carotid ultrasounds of the left internal carotid artery every 6 months to follow the progress of the moderate stenosis. He also should be maintained on one aspirin a day.

53 a) Recurrence of cancer; radiation fibrosis leading to entrapment of the trigeminal nerve or its vascular supply, resulting in trigeminal neuralgia; osteoradionecrosis (in some cases successfully treated with hyperbaric oxygen).

b) An enhancing mass lesion expanding and destroying the body and ramus of the left mandible.

54-55 a) Concussion, basilar/occipital skull fracture, and traumatic subarachnoid hemorrhage (seen along the tentorium). Note the value of bone windows in this case: the fracture is not seen with soft tissue windows.

56 a) Postconcussion syndrome.

b) Yes. Mild problems with verbal memory, trouble with sequencing tasks, mental inflexibility, and decreased right motor function suggest left frontotemporal dysfunction.

57-58 a) The association of neck pain after trauma, weakness with reflex changes in C5-6 myotomes, and C6 sensory changes strongly suggest a cervical radiculopathy. Causes in this setting could include: root contusion or avulsion, compression by bone fragment or disc herniation, extra-axial collection of blood (epidural or subdural hematoma of spinal canal), or intra-axial injury (eg, hematomyelia). The last is less likely given the absence of myelopathic signs in the lower extremities and trunk.

b) The symptoms suggest transient ischemia. Mechanical compromise of the arteries involved must be considered, such as by distortion of the vertebral artery foramen within the transverse processes of the cervical spine.

c) Obviously, a more sensitive imaging modality of the cervical spine is in order. While MR imaging has high resolution and visualizes a variety of soft tissue densities (including disc material) very well, it does not show bone well. CT scan following myelography is probably the test of choice and is shown.

d) There is an unstable fracture through the pedicles, bilaterally, also entering the left transverse process, distorting the vertebral artery foramen. The transient ischemic symptoms probably resulted from this distortion.

59 a) Notalgia paresthetica. This condition is caused by myofascial irritation of the dorsal sensory branches of upper thoracic nerve roots.

60 a) Optic neuritis.

b) False. Oral adrenocorticosteroid therapy has not been shown to be helpful and is also associated with an increased risk of optic neuritis occurring on the opposite side.

61 a) Meralgia paraesthetica. This is caused by compression or irritation at the level of the inguinal ligament of the lateral cutaneous nerve of the thigh.

62 a) Replacement of C3 and C4 by metastatic cancer.

b) Metastases to the skull base or meninges affecting cranial nerves IX and X should be considered most likely.

63-64 a) All are true. White matter deterioration accounts for these symptoms. Seizures are more likely to be of cortical origin.

65 a) Heavy smoking, chronic rhinitis, and chronic sinusitis are the most frequent causes of microsmia, which also can be noted in diabetic patients when they are examined for it. Head trauma may sever olfactory receptor cells as they pass through the cribriform plate. Recognized causes of anosmia are olfactory groove meningiomas; Alzheimer's disease; Parkinson's disease; vincristine neurotoxicity; and B_{12}, folate, and zinc deficiency.

b) Zinc deficiency. Supplementation resulted in normal olfaction within 3 weeks.

66 a) Meningioma of the falx cerebri. Curiously, her neuropsychiatric symptoms were reversed by resection of this tumor.

67 a) L4-5 disc herniation centrally.

68 a) Right middle cerebral artery infarction.

69-71 a) The most common cause is simply that one or both parents have a normally large head, as in this case. However, pathologic causes of a large head include ventricular hydrocephalus, Alexander's disease, Canavan's disease, and Tay-Sachs disease.

b) Since this is the area of the largest muscles of the body, proximal muscle weakness is most often due to a primary muscle problem (myopathic). Also, neuropathic disorders affect the longest nerves first and are therefore more likely to produce distal weakness.

c) The classic cause of tibial bowing and other skeletal changes such as "rachitic rosary" of rib costochondral junctions is rickets. Worldwide, this is most often the result of dietary deficiency of vitamin D with or without additional influence of sunlight deprivation. Exposure to sunlight is required for the conversion of 7-dehydrocholesterol to previtamin D. In developed countries this step is bypassed by widespread dietary supplementation with vitamin D_3, so dietary rickets is rare.

d) This is a case of X-linked nephrogenic hypophosphatemia

(also called familial hypophosphatemic rickets). In this condition males are often more affected than females, but variable or incomplete penetrance is the rule. Therefore, establishing the pattern of inheritance can be difficult, and the proband may be one of the only seriously affected family members. The kidney is the site of conversion of 25-hydroxycholecalciferol (25-OH-D$_3$) to 1,25-dihydroxycholecalciferol (1,25(OH)$_2$D$_3$), which is in part regulated by serum phosphate levels. Ordinarily, serum phosphate is lowered by parathyroid hormone and serves as a stimulus for this conversion. Because individuals with this syndrome lose large amounts of phosphate from the kidney, the amount of 1,25(OH)$_2$D$_3$ that they produce is insufficient to promote normal bone mineralization, resulting in rachitic bone change. Low phosphate also means low energy (ATP) reserves in muscle.

e) Formerly, so-called "vitamin D–resistant" syndromes were treated with dietary vitamin D in extremely high doses, leading to ectopic calcium deposition, including nephrolithiasis and basal ganglia calcifications. More recently, the active form of dihydroxycholecalciferol is available in an oral dosing form, thus bypassing the liver for conversion to 25-OH-D$_3$ and the subsequent renal conversion to 1,25(OH)$_2$D$_3$. Parathyroid hormone, therefore, is not called out and ectopic calcium deposition is largely avoided. In addition, large amounts of oral phosphate (as solutions of sodium phosphate) are given to keep up with decreased gut absorption and decreased renal tubular reabsorption. Overall, the prognosis for normal growth and strength is excellent if the condition is recognized in early childhood.

72 a) An arteriovenous malformation.

b) Intractable seizures or recurrent bleeding episodes.

c) All of the above.

73 a) Herpes simplex encephalitis.

b) Statements 1) and 3) are true.

74-76 a) Motor neuron disease.

b) The absence of inflammation and the presence of scattered atrophic fibers with fiber-type grouping are indicative of motor neuron disease.

77 a) Acute denervation (fibrillations, positive sharp waves) and chronic partial denervation (giant compound muscle action potentials) in the gastrocnemius muscle only.

b) Benign focal amyotrophy.

78 a) Subdural hematoma in this patient with a preexisting asymptomatic subarachnoid cyst.

79-80 a) A right cerebellar mass lesion subsequently proven pathologically to be an astrocytoma.

b) This mass is associated with considerable edema and may cause either acute obstructive hydrocephalus or upward herniation of the cerebellum, both of which may be fatal.

81 a) No.

b) A transient ischemic event.

c) An echocardiogram should be performed to rule out an embolism from chronic atrial fibrillation.

82-83 a) Ninety percent stenosis of the right internal carotid artery.

b) Endarterectomy followed by aspirin antiplatelet therapy is the current recommendation for carotid stenoses in excess of 70% defined by angiogram.

84 a) Fasciculations are spontaneous discharges of the motor unit which have been shown to originate anywhere in the axon from hillock to terminal branches.

b) In the absence of weakness or atrophy, fasciculations are considered benign and do not herald serious pathology.

c) While none are absolutely necessary, an MR scan of the spine for compressive lesions of cervical and/or lumbar roots, a serum creatine kinase (elevated in polymyositis and some instances of motor neuron disease, both of which may evidence fasciculations clinically along with weakness), and electromyographic testing for signs of acute denervation or myopathy may be considered.

85 a) Dementia of the Alzheimer type.

b) Anosmia or microsmia were probably complicating the course of his Alzheimer's disease.

86 a) Chiari malformation with associated syrinx and ventriculomegaly.

b) No. This is a congenital condition.

87 a) Overall morbidity is improved by resection of a solitary metastasis. If a solitary metastasis is surgically accessible, consideration of resection should be made. Mental status change is one of the most common presenting symptoms, although other signs may be found in a careful examination.

88 a) Pseudodementia. Hysteria would be extremely unusual in this age group.

89-90 a) Dorsal lipomatosis. This can occur spontaneously or in response to steroid treatment. Note the extremely high-intensity signal that fat produces even in T1-weighted images.

91 a) Probable dissection of the internal carotid artery.

b) Trauma and fibromuscular dysplasia.

92-95 a) Parkinson's disease with a hemiparetic presentation, expanding mass lesion in the left hemisphere, and communicating hydrocephalus need to be considered.

b) A CT or MR scan of the brain.

c) Panventriculomegaly is striking in this circumstance and strongly suggests the diagnosis of communicating hydrocephalus.

d) A lumbar puncture.

e) Chronic meningitis often produces high CSF total protein, hypoglycorrhachia, and mononuclear pleocytosis, and can be under normal CSF pressure.

f) Yes.

g) Fifty percent of cases occur in patients without any obvious reason for immunosuppression.

96 a) Dementia of the Alzheimer type.

97 a) Subarachnoid hemorrhage (note the "ground glass" density within the subarachnoid spaces).

b) 1) True. The CT scan should always be obtained at the time that suggestive clinical events occur. The diagnostic yield of a CT scan will diminish with each passing day thereafter.

2) False. The case-fatality rate still approaches 60%.

3) False.

4) True. The difference between these two entities is that surgery is not generally indicated for traumatic subarachnoid hemorrhage.

98 a) Right frontal spike discharge consistent with frontal lobe epilepsy.

b) Carbamazepine.

99 a) Ocular myasthenia gravis.

b) A tensilon test.

100 a) Although subarachnoid hemorrhage can occur during sexual intercourse, only one in twenty coital or orgasmic headaches is due to a malignant cause. Most will be due to a form of migraine called "benign coital cephalgia." If recurrent, like other forms of exercise-induced headache, this may be responsive to treatment with indomethacin.

b) The ominous cause to be considered is subarachnoid hemorrhage, most often from a saccular aneurysm in or near the circle of Willis.

c) A CT scan of the brain should be done (whenever possible) prior to cerebrospinal fluid examination. Even with a normal neurologic examination, space-occupying lesions or incipient hydrocephalus could make lumbar puncture risky or unnecessary.

d) The decreasing cell counts from Tube 1 to Tube 2, normal opening pressure, normal protein and glucose, lack of inflammatory response, and lack of xanthochromia all favor traumatic tap. However, one cannot totally exclude the possibility that a traumatic tap has obscured a small sentinel subarachnoid hemorrhage.

e) Angiography has grown safer with newer methods, but still carries a small percentage risk of dire consequences, including stroke and death. In this case, patient and physician agreed not to proceed to angiography, and 2 weeks later the patient succumbed to a grade IV subarachnoid hemorrhage. A lawsuit was filed.

101-102 a) Epilepsia partialis continua (focal motor status epilepticus).

b) Parasagittal infarction consistent with cerebral venous thrombosis.

103 a) Miller Fisher variant of Guillain-Barré syndrome (MFS).

b) Bilateral brachial plexus neuropathy complicating MFS.

104 a) All are likely. Stereotaxic biopsy revealed purulence under pressure. Cultures were positive for a *Fusobacterium* species, usually an enteric organism. No primary infection was identified. The patient recovered completely following long-term intravenous antibiotic treatment.

105 a) Absence of the left vertebral artery and marked stenosis of the midportion of the basilar artery.

b) Definitely not. He is certainly at an increased risk of progressive basilar artery occlusion leading to a major brainstem stroke, locked-in syndrome, or sudden death.

106 a) Inclusion body myositis. Note that rimmed vacuoles within muscle fibers are typically associated with this disorder.

b) Fibrillations, positive sharp waves, complex repetitive discharges, and high-amplitude polyphasic potentials, with increased recruitment at submaximal voluntary contraction of the muscle.

c) False.

107 a) In individuals with chronic cirrhosis due to alcohol, pathologic vascular (variceal) shunts may evolve whereby materials absorbed from the gut can bypass the liver and go directly to the brain and periphery. In such cases, liver function panels may not be abnormal, but serum ammonia and CSF glutamine may be elevated. Acute delirium ("hepatic encephalopathy") may result following a large protein-rich meal.

b) *Abulia* is a term that describes this man's mental status change, indicating a withdrawn, apathetic, bradyphrenic state such as was formerly achieved by prefrontal leukotomy procedures. In this case, a hemorrhagic infarction of the right frontal lobe was responsible.

c) He experienced a partial complex seizure, probably originating in the right frontal area, causing aversive movements of the head, eyes, and contralateral hand and arm.

108 a) Subdural hematoma, with acute bleeding into a chronic hematoma.

b) Subdural hematomas are crescentic and may cross suture lines. Acute subdural hematomas are hyperdense at first, but will be isodense and then hypodense as they become chronic. Occasionally they may separate into layers of density as shown. Epidural hematomas are biconvex, hyperdense in appearance, and most often found in association with a skull fracture over the middle meningeal artery, and do not cross suture lines.

109 a) Torsade de pointes. The possibility of a quinidine-induced sudden-death episode should always be considered when syncope has occurred in patients taking this medication.

110-111 a) Myopathy.

b) Start steroid treatment and obtain a right quadriceps

muscle biopsy. Initiating treatment may be lifesaving if respiratory embarrassment, which occurs in some instances of this disorder, is avoided.

   c) Childhood polymyositis.

112 a) All of the above.

113 a) Olivopontocerebellar atrophy.

114 a) A thalamic stereotactic radio-frequency lesion. While this may easily be a lacunar infarct, in fact, it was the result of successful neurosurgery for intractable tremor. No sensory deficits were induced by this iatrogenic lesion.

115-116 a) Extensive left hemispheric encephalomalacia with islands of normal brain anteriorly and posteriorly are seen on CT, and diminished amplitudes of normal waveforms over the left hemisphere are recorded on EEG. Remarkably, this woman presumably acquired this extensive lesion at age 9 but now is neurologically normal (including language and right-sided motor functions), testifying to the plasticity of the young nervous system.

117 a) A left parietal infarct.

   b) Impaired reading, writing, and calculating might accompany the inability to accurately produce individually named fingers of the right hand to command (finger agnosia). These four signs are the quadrad of Gerstmann's syndrome, which is rarely, if ever, found in isolation, but more frequently is accompanied by a right hemiparesis and hemihypesthesia.

118 a) Enlargement of the ventricular system with a frontal span exceeding 42 mm in this clinical setting is suggestive of normal pressure (communicating) hydrocephalus.

   b) A lumbar puncture removing 25 cc of cerebrospinal fluid may improve memory, gait, or continence. This patient's gait improved dramatically and all of her complaints resolved after ventriculoperitoneal shunting.

119 a) Malingering. By chance alone, the subject should achieve at least 9 correct answers. Purposeful errors indicate intact olfaction.

120 a) Mass lesions in the cerebellopontine angle, posterior fossa arteriovenous malformation, and multiple sclerosis need to be considered.

b) T2-weighted MR images show multiple white-matter lesions most consistent with multiple sclerosis.

121 a) Chiari malformation. The localizing value of downbeat nystagmus is for the region of the cervicocranial junction, so all of these choices could cause it. The exact mechanism for the phenytoin and lithium effects is not known. Other types of nystagmus can be seen as one element in a syndrome of paraneoplastic cerebellar degeneration, although ataxia is a more frequent manifestation.

122 a) Polymyositis.

b) Fibrillations and positive sharp waves (usually signs of neurogenic denervation) may be observed during needle electromyographic testing of patients with inflammatory myopathies due to functional disconnection of muscle fibers remote from nerve terminals. They are normally recruited to discharge with others of the motor unit by transmembrane depolarization of juxtaposed fibers, one of which is in contact with the nerve terminal. Inflammatory injury to interposed muscle fibers "denervates" other fibers, which then fibrillate.

123-126 a) A hypothalamic lesion may yield behavior changes including goal-directed violence, polydipsia, and polyuria.

b) Frontotemporal atrophy.

c) Mild bifrontal slowing.

d) All of the above.

e) Pick's disease. The abnormal inclusion (Pick) body is the hallmark of this disease and is most commonly encountered in the temporal lobe neocortex, but can be missed if biopsy material is taken from the frontal lobe.

127 a) Spike and wave discharges (5/s) during which the patient was noted to stare and be unresponsive.

b) Typical absence epilepsy occurs in children 4 to 8 years of age and is associated with a 3/s spike and wave pattern on EEG. The condition is inherited in an autosomal dominant pattern with age-dependent penetrance. Absences typically last 5 to 10 seconds and may occur hundreds of times a day without aura or postictal confusion.

Notes

Notes

Notes

Notes

Notes

Notes

Notes